MW01633862

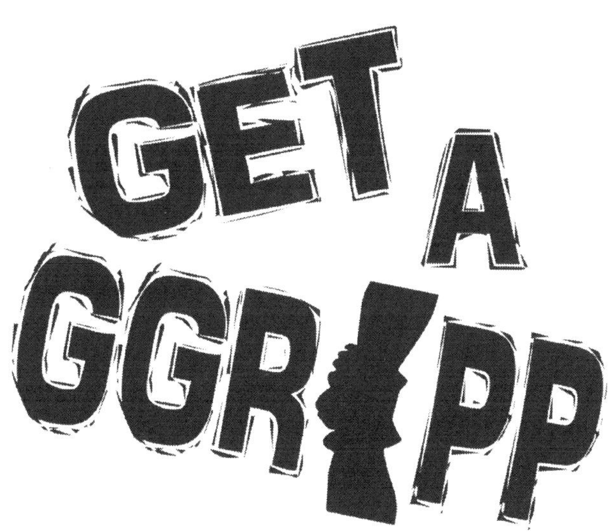

THE HEALTH AND WELLNESS MOVEMENT ROOTED IN BLACK CULTURAL TRADITIONS

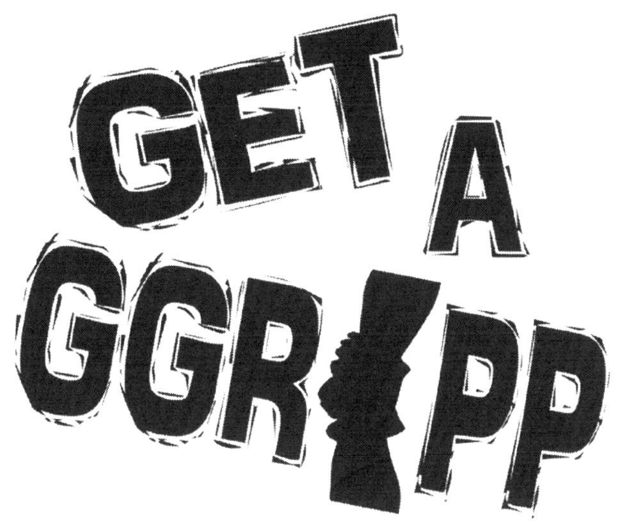

THE HEALTH AND WELLNESS MOVEMENT ROOTED IN BLACK CULTURAL TRADITIONS

BY TANYA LEAKE
FOUNDER, EMBODY WELL

ISBN-10: 0692939229
ISBN-13: 978-0692939222 (EmBODY WELL)

©2017 EmBODY WELL. All Rights Reserved.
First Printing: 2017. The editorial arrangement, analysis, and professional commentary are subject to this copyright notice. No portion of this book may be copied, retransmitted, reposted, duplicated, or otherwise used without the express written approval of the author, except by reviewers who may quote brief excerpts in connection with a review. Brief quotations may be used in reviews prepared for inclusion in a magazine, newspaper, or for broadcast.

United States laws and regulations are public domain and not subject to copyright. Any unauthorized copying, reproduction, translation, or distribution of any part of this material without permission by the author is prohibited and against the law.

Disclaimer and Terms of Use: This book presents information based upon the research and personal experiences of the author. It is not intended to be a substitute for a professional consultation with a physician or other health-care provider. If you have a condition that requires medical advice, the publisher and author urge you to consult a competent health-care professional.

Your reliance upon information and content obtained by you at or through this publication is solely at your own risk. EmBODY WELL and the author assume no liability or responsibility for damage or injury to you, other persons, or property arising from any use of any product, information, idea, or instruction contained in the content or services provided to you through this book. Reliance upon information contained in this material is solely at the reader's own risk. The author has no financial interest in and receive no compensation from non-EmBODY WELL manufacturers of products or websites mentioned in this book.

For my dear friend Magnus: memories of you will always bring me joy while the unexpected and unnecessary loss of you will always be a reminder of the critical need for community health awareness, support and prevention.

My vision board reads…" Start a Movement."

Here it is, and I pray it catches on…

Preface

Magnus: "I went by the health fair today, Tanya. They took my blood pressure and said it was really high."

Me: "How high was it, Magnus?"

As I was finishing this book, I had the painful experience of finding my good friend Magnus Christon dead on the floor of his bathroom, suddenly and unexpectedly at the age of 50. The cause of death? "Hypertensive cardiovascular heart disease." For some, that meant *heart* failure. For me, it meant what felt like *my* failure. Months before, he told me he had gotten his blood pressure tested and that it was *really* high. He and I discussed the fact that blood pressure was a "silent killer," especially in Our community. Although I kept pushing him to get to a doctor to get it treated, he kept telling me he was between doctors, trying to find one, so I knew that it was *not* being treated. Shortly before his death, he shared with me that he had not been feeling well, that he had something he "could not shake." Around the same time (as I later learned), he had also shared with other friends and colleagues, specific, somewhat alarming symptoms. My wish/regret? That We could have put the pieces together as a community, as *his* community of family and friends, and provided the needed support to ultimately prevent his unnecessary death.

My friend Magnus was a caring, community-centered person who had done so much for so many. Even with so many contributions, I still regret that Magnus left us too early with too much *untapped potential.* Among other things, **GET A GGRiPP** is an opportunity to somewhat soothe my regrets and make Magnus proud. **GET A GGRiPP** practices the same caring, community-centered approach that he did. And my hope for **GET A GGRiPP** is that it will be a tool (and a movement) to enable Our community to *tap its full potential* with the help of improved community health awareness, support and prevention.

Why read this book?
Because you care…about yourself, your family, your village, your community…and because you care enough to be part of a movement that can change how you live and the world you live in.

"The future of the race depends on the conservation of its health."
Booker T. Washington

There has been and continues to be a lot of discussion about what the Black community in America needs: the need for progress, the need for justice, the need for protection from injustice, the need for economic and social advancement, the need for community empowerment. The problem with the discussion to date is that it has largely ignored the link between these larger needs and the need for good health.

The link between "the health of the race and racial progress" is not new…There are historical examples of efforts to *address the health needs* of the Black community *as a vehicle to broader community empowerment.*

In 1913, Booker T. Washington said, "Without health, […] it will be impossible for [Black people] to have permanent success in business, in property getting, in acquiring education, or to show other evidences of progress." He "viewed the poor health status of Black Americans as an obstacle to economic progress."[1] These beliefs led to his founding of National Health Improvement Week in 1915. National Health Improvement Week evolved into National Negro Health Week (NNHW) which then "evolved into "a comprehensive year-round program, […] entitled the National

---

[1] Quinn, Sandra Crouse and Thomas, Stephen B. "The National Negro Health Week, 1915 to 1951: A Descriptive Account." Minority Health Today, Vol 2, Num 3, (Mar/Apr 2001): 44

Negro Health Movement." This program, his legacy and the goal of improving black health status as a stepping stone to progress in other areas continued until 1951 - when its then supporting organization, the US Office of Negro Health Work, was officially dismantled.[2]

Taking up the mantle in 1966, the Black Panthers identified Black community health as a foundational social justice issue. The Black Panthers called for and established free community health care clinics as part of their core activities, effectively declaring that the health of the Black community was a critical component to achieving broader social justice. And, in 1972, "health was formally added as the sixth point" of the Black Panthers Ten Point Program guiding document.[3] This sixth point not only outlined the need for treatment facilities (community clinics) to address diseases that were the "result of [Black] oppression" but also the need for broader "preventative medical programs to guarantee [the Black community's] future survival."[4]

NNHW and the Black Panther's Ten Point Program are only two examples of previous community-based movements focused on improving health yet whose ultimate mission was/is improving the broader status of the Black community. The idea is not new and the potential is great given that Black health sits on such a strong physical and mental foundation. Physically, our assets have been consistently leveraged to others' benefit, as slaves, athletes, and even soldiers; as early as 1924, military studies showed that the percentage of those considered militarily fit and qualified among Black registrants was consistently higher than the percent of

---

[2] Quinn and Thomas, "The National Negro Health Week, 1915 to 1951: A Descriptive Account": 48

[3] Bassett, M. T. (2016). Beyond Berets: The Black Panthers as Health Activists. American Journal of Public Health, 106(10): 1741–1743. *http://doi.org/10.2105/AJPH.2016.303412*

[4] "History of the Black Panther Party: Black Panther Party Platform and Program." The Black Panther. (23 Nov 1967):3. *https://web.stanford.edu/group/blackpanthers/history.shtml*

militarily fit and qualified among White registrants.[5] Mentally, we have shown incredible strength, demonstrating a consistent and seemingly infinite hope for progress in the face of evidence to the contrary. As concluded by the authors of a descriptive account of NNHW, "if today's campaigns can draw upon the racial pride and strengths and assets within the Black community, we will enhance likelihood of success."

Enter **GET A GGRiPP**…

"It is possible for you to get a grip on the thing
that used to have a grip on you."
TD Jakes

GET A GGRiPP is what seems like the natural evolution of my experience working publicly and privately in and around Black community health and wellness. I committed myself to a full-time career in health and wellness because of a personal passion for the health of my community, which has affected and continues to affect me directly. I have watched as "my village," family, friends (like Magnus), friends of friends, and so on, have suffered with various acute and chronic mental and physical health conditions and diseases that are treatable and/or preventable. I have mourned the loss of strong and promising community supporters, educators, and leaders due to health issues. This led me to ask myself what is needed (missing) in the health and wellness industry today, especially when it comes to serving the needs of a Black population whose health outcomes still lag their white counterparts? In other words, how can we "get a grip on the thing that has a grip on us?"

---

[5] Jackson, Algernon B. "The Need for Health Education Among Negroes." Opportunity: Journal of Negro Life, (Aug, 1924) *http://health-equity.lib.umd.edu/2/1/need_of_health_education.pdf*

My conclusion? What is needed (missing) in the h
wellness industry for the Black community is "targetin
occurred to me mostly as a result of my experience as African
American Campaign Coordinator" for the Network for a Healthy
California (a previous program of the California Department of
Public Health).

The "Empowerment Agenda" for the African-American
Campaign reads as follows[6]:

"The Network for a Healthy California – African American
Campaign is one of five targeted campaigns established to address
[…] health disparities by empowering low-income African
American families to make healthy food choices and be physically
active through education, advocacy and community
empowerment."

The African American Campaign operated based on the belief that
"strategies, programs and policies specifically designed for and
targeting African Americans" was not only needed but "essential"
in "building healthy African American communities." That
acknowledging the unique experience of Blacks in America, i.e.
being "culturally competent," was critical to the success of an
overall strategy to improve the health of Black communities in
America. This cultural competence meant not only incorporating
"slave religious and cultural traditions [that] played a particularly
important role in helping slaves survive the harshness and misery
of life under slavery"[7] but also, as I defined it, acknowledging Black

---

[6] "Advocating for the Health of Our Communities: Consumer Empowerment Agenda of
the Network for a Healthy California – African American Campaign Advisory Council."
(Jun   2008)   _http://cachampionsforchange.cdph.ca.gov/Documents/Join   the
Movement/Take Action in Your Community/BRO-191 JUN 2008.pdf_

[7] Mintz, Steven and Stauffer, John. The Problem of Evil: Slavery, Freedom and the
Ambiguities of American Reform. Univ of Massachusetts Press (2007): 28.

American psychology, attitudes and expectations as a result of life under and after slavery.

After over a year as the lead for the African American Campaign, I was told that the plan was to merge the five targeted campaigns into a single "minority" campaign (reason given? similar to the reasoning for the dismantling of the Office of Negro Health – *integration*). Based on what I had seen and the work I had done in the role, I knew that was a bad idea. It was, always has been and still is a bad idea to "dilute" (and ignore) cultural distinctions among "minority" cultures. It was then that I began to fully realize what was "needed." In response to news of the plan to "merge," I put together what I called my "culture in context" presentation. It was designed to provide an overview of the African American Campaign and describe how Black culture could and should be applied in context to achieve the Campaign's goals. Specifically, it detailed four points of "Black cultural competence"[8] and my recommendations for applying them in the context of the Campaign. I emphasized that the unique culture of the Black community grew out of oppression and was rooted in the legacy of slavery. Like the founders of NNHW and the Black Panther Ten Point Program, I knew that **health empowerment** goals **could also be a means to overall empowerment** of the Black community; however, I also knew it could only succeed with a program that acknowledged the community's unique cultural roots. This was the beginning of **GET A GGRiPP**.

Of all the health and wellness plans and solutions I explored leading up to **GET A GGRiPP**, I could not find what I considered a "culturally competent" and <u>complete</u> health and wellness plan specifically designed for, targeted at and a reflection of the Black community. **GET A GGRiPP** is thus the first-of-its-kind "culturally competent," *culturally-rooted*, <u>complete</u> health and wellness plan. It provides the missing piece I was looking for in

---

[8] Four points of "Blacl cultural competence:" 1) history of oppression and trauma ; 2) mis/dis-trust for outsiders; 3) focus on difference; 4) distinct culture

other solutions, "cultural targeting." **GET A GGRiPP** combines my health and wellness experience as a fitness instructor and health educator with my personal knowledge of and research on Black cultural traditions. Like the NNHW, the Black Panther Ten Point Program and other movements before it, **GET A GGRiPP** is intended not only to create a new tradition of health rooted in our historical cultural traditions, but also unite us around a common goal that inspires us beyond our need for a "clean bill of health." Rooted specifically in the Black cultural traditions of dance, music, comedy, food and faith, **GET A GGRiPP** is the "for us, by us" health and wellness movement, making health and wellness accessible and easy "for us" to succeed because it is, ultimately, "by us."

GET A…

GRUB: Get That Green

GROOVE: Show Your Roots

RELEASE: Bust a Gut

i

POWER: Soul Train

PEACE: Breathe Inside Out

Acknowledgments

Thanks to the following folks without whom **GET A GGRiPP** would not have seen the light of day...

Carol, for pushing me to the starting line.

JAG, Al-b, J-Boogie, and Nnek for reviews and edits that moved me to the finish line.

Daddy and Ma Bev, for staying up with me, listening to late night rantings and readings.

Mikai, JJ, Mackenzie, Cameron, and CJ, for giving me 5 more reasons to want a healthier, stronger community.

Derrick of DonLeoDesigns, book designer extraordinaire, for rolling with the lunatic timeframes and constant "special" requests.

My friends, clients and faithful students for always being supportive, willing guinea pigs and inspiring me every day.

INTRO

Wellness MATTERS.

The future of Our community depends on Us achieving health and wellness. Yet, given the disparities We consistently see in Our health outcomes, it is apparent that "getting a grip on what has a grip on Us" is a unique challenge in the Black community. Could it be that not "seeing" Ourselves in the solutions that exist today directly impacts Our success in eliminating disparities and achieving health and wellness? Could the challenge be that We are not targeted, or "represented," in today's health and wellness solutions? The future of the community is dependent on us finding a solution to this challenge.

GET A GGRiPP represents that solution. **GET A GGRiPP** represents a new approach to wellness for Black people of African descent, a wellness plan rooted in Afro cultural traditions, a wellness solution targeted at the unique needs of the Black community, a wellness movement designed to use health empowerment as a vehicle to broader community empowerment. **GET A GGRiPP** applies Our cultural history of "changing the game" to change the game of wellness. We can succeed in wellness *and* help Our communities succeed by returning to Our roots with a "culturally authentic" wellness solution. Unlocking wellness is possible when the keys are easy, accessible and fun. It is the "for Us, by Us" wellness solution that makes health and wellness easy, accessible and fun (it feels natural and good "for Us") because it is rooted in Black cultural traditions (already done "by Us"). It is the solution that will finally enable Us to "**GET A GGRiPP**" on Our health…and our future!

A. WELLNESS Matters:
What is GET A GGRiPP?

GET A GGRiPP is a movement, a message *and* a prescription for Our health... The message? We need to "get a grip" on Our health. The prescription? Follow the steps of the acronym's 5 easy to remember and relatable healthy lifestyle elements, namely:

GET A...

GRUB: Get That Green

GROOVE: Show Your Roots

RELEASE: Bust a Gut

i

POWER: Soul Train

PEACE: Breathe Inside Out

GET A GGRiPP's 5 healthy lifestyle elements are rooted in Our culturally significant and uniquely creative approaches to Our food and eating, Our dance and music, Our laughter and humor, and Our strength, faith and hope.

GET A GGRiPP (2G's, 1R, 2P's) is also a movement for Us, on two levels. First, it represents a movement for Us to "get a grip" on Our health, wellness and overall wellbeing. Once Our wellbeing is taken care of, We can "get a grip" on moving Our community forward in other ways. Remember, **GET A GGRiPP** is not just about getting a grip on Our physical health; it's about getting a grip on the physical, mental, emotional, economic AND political "health" of Our community. The main principle of **GET A GGRiPP** is that We will only truly be able to take care of Ourselves (and meet Our larger needs as a community) once We take care of Ourselves (by meeting the health needs of Our community).

How does **GET A GGRiPP** do all this? Three key ways…

1. Cultural Targeting

Based on my training and practical experience working with client behavior change as a health coach and fitness instructor, I have learned that success in healthy lifestyle change is the result of starting with small, easy steps and gradually making additional small changes. It is also common knowledge in the health and wellness industry that, for wellness to be attainable, it must be accessible. Rooted in cultural norms that make them easy and accessible to Us, **GET A GGRiPP**'s healthy lifestyle elements are targeted to Our *specific* health and wellness needs. That is, to ensure success, all elements:

- "TAKE IT BACK" (are culturally rooted in Our history) - all elements are rooted in a Black cultural activity We have historically done in a way uniquely Ours.

- "KEEP IT SIMPLE" (are culturally easy) - all elements are based on a healthy version of an activity that is "easy" for Us because We (likely) do (or can do) them.

- "BRING IT HOME" (are culturally relevant) - all elements serve the *unique* needs and challenges of Our community from a wellness perspective. (see #2 below)

2. Mind AND Body Benefits (MBB)

What remains after Our long history of slavery and oppression runs deep and, over time, has resulted in significant distress. Uniquely Ours, this distress exists in both Our minds and Our bodies and, given its depth, is difficult to resolve and release. That is why all **GET A GGRiPP** elements benefit both mind and body. The approach that will benefit Us most provides both Mind AND Body Benefits (MBB). You will see references to MBB throughout this book. As you will see, every element of **GET A**

GGRiPP incorporates MBB, acknowledging and leveraging the importance and significance of the mind-body connection in achieving wellness…*especially and specifically for Us.* By taking a holistic, MBB approach, **GET A GGRiPP** becomes a <u>complete cultural wellness solution</u>, incorporating elements in a way that no current health and fitness plan provides today.

3. A Movement in "Common-unity"

Last but certainly not least, the ultimate goal of **GET A GGRiPP** is more than a *healthier* community; it is a *stronger* community. **GET A GGRiPP** is not just a health and wellness plan, it is a community movement. For Us, health and wellness has been and will always be influenced and impacted by Our social circles. By *uniting* Us around cultural activities that reinforce Our *common* roots, **GET A GGRiPP** builds "common-unity" that empowers Us to make progress in more than just health. Each of the elements of **GET A GGRiPP** can (and should) be shared and celebrated with Our family and friends and in Our social and professional circles. As We do this, We build the health, strength and "common-unity" of and in Our communities.

ONE MORE THING!

A NOTE ABOUT "THESE THREE WORDS" AND *US*: You'll notice through this book that "these three words," "Us", "We", and "Our" are capitalized. Capitalization serves two purposes. First, when We see and read these three words throughout the book, We are reminded that **GET A GGRiPP** is about community. It is a constant reminder that **GET A GGRiPP** elements are done best together - in community and for the benefit of "common-unity." The secondary goal of capitalization is to refer to Ourselves "properly." Capitalization makes these 3 words proper nouns. Because proper nouns refer to a particular thing or a one-of-a-kind item, using these three words as proper nouns reminds Us that We are one-of-a-kind and special. It is intended to instill pride, respect, esteem, love and "common-unity." When We see these three "short and simple" words, We will be reminded to be "sweet and kind" to ourselves and one another.

B. On the GET A GGRiPP TIP: How do I GET A GGRiPP?

How does it work? All the details you need to get started with **GET A GGRiPP** are on the following pages! Find a buddy (or 2 or 3 or 4 or more!) and **GET A GGRiPP** together! Remember, this is a "Common-Unity" affair! **GET A GGRiPP** is easy and accessible to everyone in Our community, from any income level and any location. There is no special equipment or gym membership required! The sooner We begin learning, practicing and sharing the elements of **GET A GGRiPP**, the sooner We'll be healthier, seeing MBB and making a difference in Our common-unity! Ready, SET…

…WAIT, one more thing! Pay attention to the TIPs for each **GET A GGRiPP** healthy lifestyle element. TIPs stand for (T)ype, (I)ntensity and (P)ointer(s). "Type" describes the element at its most basic, simple AND culturally relevant. "Intensity" describes the various levels you can incorporate the element into your daily life. If you are new to an element, start with the low intensity. More experienced? Challenge yourself with a higher intensity! …or start anywhere in between that works for you. "Pointers" are just that...recommendations and tips to help you **GET A GGRiPP**! The next chapters describe each of the 5 healthy lifestyle elements of **GET A GGRiPP** in detail.

Disclaimer: Consult your medical professional about the healthy lifestyle elements of **GET A GGRiPP** to determine what levels for each element are appropriate for you.

I. GRUB: Get That Green

> "True soul food is what you feed your body when
> you treat it like a temple."
> Tanya Leake

A.   GRUB Matters

Everyone needs food to survive. However, good health and wellness is about more than surviving, it's about thriving. It is consensus in the health and wellness community that eating well can be a bigger contributor to your overall health than "exercising well." Big health improvements can come from small changes in nutrition and eating habits. Because of this, many health advocates encourage vegetarian or vegan lifestyles as the best approach to eating for good health. However, vegetarians and vegan lifestyles define eating habits based on what not to do instead of what to do. Given Our history of expropriation (things being taken from Us) and deprivation (things being denied Us), **a healthier** *(and easier)* **approach for Us is to focus on what to include, not what to exclude**. I have coined the term "vegetablarian" to reflect just that. A vegetablarian lifestyle is defined as a lifestyle that *includes* lots of vegetables. By changing my focus in this way, I have achieved health and wellness without *necessarily* (it's always my option) excluding so-called "unhealthy" foods.

Why focus on vegetables? As a health coach and founder of the "vegetablarian" movement, I know that vegetables line up well against many of the major health challenges We disproportionately suffer from: they are low in calories (to combat obesity), they are low in sugar (to combat diabetes), they are low in sodium (to combat high blood pressure and heart disease); they are high in water, fiber, vitamins, minerals and disease-fighting (phyto-)

nutrients (to combat physical dis-ease deficiencies and mental distress).[9] Studies have shown that eating well, especially consuming whole (not packaged, processed or fast) foods like vegetables, supports good health AND can help prevent disease. Both the US Department of Agriculture and Harvard University recommend making half of every plate vegetables and/or fruits[10] (although mostly vegetables[11]). In fact, eating whole foods like vegetables has been proven to support not only a healthy body but also a healthy *mind*. Yes! The latest research links healthy eating and whole foods to good mental health.[12] There is even an (emerging) field called Nutritional Psychiatry based on this link![13] When We GRUB well, We *feel* well, physically AND emotionally!

B.   On the GRUB TIP

So how do We **GET A GGRiPP** on Our GRUB? "Get that green." In other words, let's make eating green "a black thing!" Green, leafy vegetables that is! The fact that the food that We traditionally prepare is commonly called "soul food" means that mealtimes for Us are more than just about survival, they are "sacred."   Food has been and continues to be an integral component of Black community rituals and activities. From fixin

---

[9] "Why is it important to eat vegetables?" (12 Jan 2016) *https://www.choosemyplate.gov/vegetables-nutrients-health*

[10] "Healthy Eating Plate and Healthy Eating Pyramid." Harvard University, TH Chan School of Public Health (2011). *https://www.hsph.harvard.edu/nutritionsource/healthy-eating-plate/*

[11] "Vegetables and Fruits." Harvard University, TH Chan School of Public Health (2011). *https://www.hsph.harvard.edu/nutritionsource/what-should-you-eat/vegetables-and-fruits/*

[12] Telis, Gisela. "Can what you eat affect your mental health? New research links diet and the mind." The Washington Post (24 Mar 2014). *https://www.washingtonpost.com/national/health-science/can-what-you-eat-affect-your-mental-health-new-research-links-diet-and-the-mind/2014/03/24/c6b40876-abc0-11e3-af5f-4c56b834c4bf_story.html*

[13] Selhub, Eva. "Nutritional psychiatry: Your brain on food." Harvard Health Publications, Harvard Medical School (16 Nov 2015) *http://www.health.harvard.edu/blog/nutritional-psychiatry-your-brain-on-food-201511168626*

the "GRUB" to presentin the "GRUB" to "GRUBbin," activities around "GRUB" are a source of cultural and social pride. Given Our particular risk for disease, Our wellness is especially dependent on Us ensuring that Our "soul food" lives up to its name, not only *feeding* Our bodies but *nourishing* Our "souls" as well.

According to the Oldways African Heritage Diet, "a way of eating based on the healthy food traditions of people with African roots,"[14] the foundation of a traditional healthy diet for people of African descent is green, leafy vegetables. It's what We should GRUB on the most. PERIOD. Raw or cooked, green leafy vegetables are the major part of the **GET A GGRiPP** GRUB approach. Why green? Green, leafy vegetables are considered the kings and queens of the (vegetable) jungle, especially for Us! Remember, if We get Our GRUB on green leafy vegetables, We are focusing on the most important sources of nourishment for Our bodies and minds!!! So, **GET A GGRiPP** on GRUB and "get that green" every day!

1. (T)ype

Leafy greens...that's the focus! Get that green! It's that simple!

2. (I)ntensity

(Start) Low:

If you currently don't GRUB on a lot of vegetables, start by adding a green leafy vegetable to one of your meals daily.

(Go) High:

At the next level, make leafy green vegetables at least half (50%) of the vegetables you GRUB on. If you are already there, continue to increase the percent of green leafy vegetables on your plate every day!

---

[14] "African Heritage Diet." Oldways Preservation and Exchange Trust (2011). *http://oldwayspt.org/traditional-diets/african-heritage-diet*

3. (P)ointers

(1) The greener, the better! Color is a great indicator of the vibrancy and strength of your vegetables (especially greens) and their nutrients. Keep your greens green – don't cook them too long (and never boil them)!

(2) Try different preparations. Often, We don't like certain foods because of the way they are prepared. For green leafy vegetables, there are quite a few options: raw in smoothies (green smoothies are hot right now!) or salads, steamed, "healthy sautéed[15]," simmered in a pot or oven-roasted! Even if you cook them, feel free to set aside a few raw leaves to add as topping or garnish! Want some help? Watch EmBODY WELL's latest "GRUB and Groove" vegetablarian-cooking show which focuses *exclusively* on vegetable preparation!

(3) Start by loading your plate (1/2 full) with the "good stuff," vegetables, especially your green leafies, FIRST! That way you make sure there is plenty of room for them. In addition, if you are still hungry and want seconds, again, get that green first!

(4) Fresh and/or frozen vegetables are preferable to canned for a few reasons, namely additives in canned foods, especially sodium, as well as chemicals used in packaging, such as BPA. If you only have access to canned vegetables, rinse them before cooking to reduce the sodium and look for BPA-free packaging.

NOTE: Kale and other green leafy vegetables <u>can</u> interfere with blood thinning drugs. It is usually only a problem with sudden

---

[15] Healthy sautéing replaces traditional fats and oils with a small amount of liquid, broth, wine, juice or water to cook foods. Google "healthy saute" for more information.

changes in consumption;[16] however, if you are taking any medications, be sure to consult your health professionals about new eating habits and potential interactions with those medications.

---

[16] Begun, Rachel. "5 Common Food-Drug Interactions." Academy of Nutrition and Dietetics (9 Oct 2014). *http://www.eatright.org/resource/health/wellness/preventing-illness/common-food-drug-interactions*

ONE MORE THING!

A NOTE ABOUT WATER AND *US*: What We eat AND what We drink are equally important! As Black Americans, We are more likely to consume sugar-sweetened beverages AND are at higher risk to suffer from related conditions (obesity, diabetes, etc.).[17] Although vegetables can help Us better hydrate through food (vegetables are high in water content), nothing is better than water for hydration. In particular, We should enjoy drinking water instead of sugary beverages (like soda, sweet tea <u>and</u> juice) so that We can toast to better health!

---

[17] "Impact of Sugar-Sweetened Beverage Consumption on Black Americans' Health. A Research Brief." The African American Collaborative Obesity Research Network. (January 2011): 1.

II. GROOVE: Show Your Roots

"Hard times require furious dancing..."
Alice Walker

A.   GROOVE Matters

Cardiovascular health is more than just a notion, especially for Us. Heart disease is the #1 killer of all Americans AND We are at an even higher risk (than Our white counterparts). We are also at higher risk for contributors to heart disease, including high blood pressure, diabetes, obesity and (especially) stress.[18] Cardiovascular exercise (or cardio for short), exercising your heart, is an integral part of any disease prevention plan and a *critical* component of a Black wellness plan.

According to the US Department of Health and Human Services, the general recommendation for the amount of cardiovascular activity for adults to maintain good health is 30 minutes a day, 5 days a week (or 150 minutes weekly). This should be done at a moderate intensity (you can talk but can't sing)[19]. To lose weight or for improved health (or for children 6-17), the guideline is higher - 60 minutes a day, 5 days a week, (or 300 minutes weekly) at a moderate intensity. If you choose to exercise your heart at a higher intensity (you can't talk OR sing), you can increase the

---

[18] Leigh, J. A., Alvarez, M., & Rodriguez, C. J. (2016). "Ethnic Minorities and Coronary Heart Disease: an Update and Future Directions." Current Atherosclerosis Reports: 18(2), 9, *https://www.ncbi.nlm.nih.gov/pmc/articles/PMC4828242/*

[19] "Appendix 1. Physical Activity Guidelines for Americans." Dietary Guidelines 2015-2020, health.gov, *https://health.gov/dietaryguidelines/2015/guidelines/appendix-1/*

efficiency of your exercise (and cut your exercise time in half)! You can also choose to break the daily recommendation time into short (5-10 minute) bouts or bursts or exercise throughout the day. Studies have shown that short, frequent bursts could actually be more beneficial[20] so time is no excuse!

B. On the **GROOVE TIP**

So how do We **GET A GGRiPP** on cardio? Luckily for Us, one of Our most common culturally-rooted activities happens to be a great form of cardio! As humans, Our bodies are designed to move; as Black folks, Our bodies are designed to GROOVE! Throughout the African Diaspora, the tradition of "GROOVING" is strong. "Dance, in the African tradition, and thus in the tradition of slaves, was a part of both everyday life and special occasions."[21] John Miller Chernoff states that African peoples "do not so much observe rituals in their lives, as they ritualize their lives."[22] Dance has been part of Our survival and Our resistance: slave traders made Us dance for exercise during the Middle Passage and We used it during and after slavery as a way of maintaining a connection to Our ancestral traditions, (e.g. worship and the ring shout). Historically, it also provided Us a means of communication for self-defense and self-preservation (e.g. capoeira)[23] and We have used it as an alternative to violence and as an escape/coping mechanism (e.g. breakdancing).

---

[20] Glazer, N. L., Lyass, A., Esliger, D. W., Blease, S. J., Freedson, P. S., Massaro, J. M., … Vasan, R. S. (2013). "Sustained and Shorter Bouts of Physical Activity are Related to Cardiovascular Health." Medicine and Science in Sports and Exercise, 45(1): 109–115. *https://www.ncbi.nlm.nih.gov/pmc/articles/PMC4166425/*

[21] "African-American Culture." Wikipedia, *https://en.wikipedia.org/wiki/African-American culture - Dance*

[22] Chernoff, John Miller. African Rhythm and African Sensibility. Chicago and London: University of Chicago Press (1979): 160.

[23] "Dance, Diasporic." Encyclopedia of African-American Culture and History. Encyclopedia.com.   (August   10,   2017). http://www.encyclopedia.com/history/encyclopedias-almanacs-transcripts-and-maps/dance-diasporic

Because of Our cultural relationship to dance, it has two advantages over traditional cardio for Us. First, as a "natural" activity for Us (it is not only socially accepted, but typically socially *expected* in Our community), dance is often easier to incorporate consistently in Our daily lives (than traditional cardio). Second, given Our higher risk for mental AND physical contributors to heart disease, We need the significant added MBB of GROOVING! Studies have shown dancing is beneficial to both the mind and body. Personally, dance has always been a "grounding" influence for me; I find that when I dance, I am happier and less moody. I have also seen how GROOVING (or lack of GROOVING!) can change the mood of an entire room of Us in an instant. Want MBB? Dancing not only supports improvements in heart and blood vessel functioning, balance, flexibility and weight management, it has been linked to improvements in memory, and reductions in stress and symptoms of depression and anxiety. When We GROOVE, the way We move and the music we hear allow our bodies and minds to connect so both benefit!

According to Merriam-Webster, the definition of dance is "to move one's body rhythmically to music." When We GROOVE, We not only get the cardiovascular benefits, We also strengthen the mind-body connection as we develop comfort in Our bodies, increasing confidence and self-esteem. So, **GET A GGRiPP** on cardio, get your "natural-born" GROOVE on… and "show your roots" every day!

1. (T)ype

Dance…like no one is watching! GROOVE…what you feel! Any type of dance will do; remember, according to the definition, any movement of your body to music counts ("rhythmically" is optional). GET. YOUR. GROOVE. ON…SHOW. YOUR. ROOTS!

2. (I)ntensity

(Start) Low:

Find music that inspires you to GROOVE and do what you are "moved" to do! GROOVE intensely enough that it is difficult to sing (even though you might want to)! Keep it movin' for 5-10 minutes at a time!!![24]

(Go) High:

Raise the roof and/or get low! Raising your arms above your heart makes it *work harder*! Also, the lower you get, the harder your heart works to keep your legs strong! Jumping off the floor adds even more intensity! GROOVE enough that it is difficult to talk in complete sentences. Repeat to exhaustion! Take a little rest and start again!

3. (P)ointers

(1) Stop, look and listen for music that makes you want to move! Be constantly inspired to GROOVE!

(2) Recent studies highlight the benefits of non-exercise activity (also called NEAT) for weight management and overall health.[25] Don't restrict yourself to a single time of day. Show your roots and GROOVE at various times of the day throughout the day. To remind yourself to GROOVE, set alarms on your phone, use sticky notes or make it a habit by attaching your GROOVE to something you already do (while you brush your teeth, fix your meals) or a place you already go (your bedroom, your child's room, the den) regularly.

---

[24] DeNoon, Daniel. "Combine brief bouts of moderate exercise for health." Harvard Health Publications, Harvard Medical School (11 Sep 2013). *http://www.health.harvard.edu/blog/combine-brief-bouts-of-moderate-exercise-for-health-201309116670*

[25] Schiller, Ben. "The Spectacular Benefits of Non-Exercise: How Little Movements Add Up to a Healthier Day." Fast Company (24 Mar 2016). *https://www.fastcompany.com/3057995/the-spectacular-benefits-of-non-exercise-how-little-movements-add-up-to-a-healthier-day*

(3) You can even GROOVE while sitting! Remember, as you get your arms above your heart you can get cardiovascular benefits! And even leg or foot tapping can spark the burn! Find the right music and GROOVE something!

(4) FOR THE SISTAS: Don't let your hair spoil your GROOVE! Take advantage of the "breakdown" – multiple short bursts of exercise throughout the day - in 5-10 minutes, you can get just as much benefit and show only the roots you want to show! Be warned, once you start to GROOVE, it may be hard to stop!

(5) Get inspiration from (or just follow along with) videos. YouTube has a wide variety of dance fitness videos and styles! Or you can check out getaggripp.com/groove for a variety of EmBODY WELL dance fitness videos!

NOTE: Be sure to consult your health professionals before starting a new cardiovascular exercise program to confirm safe ranges for duration and intensity, *especially* if you have high blood pressure or diabetes.

III. RELEASE: Bust A Gut

"I love myself when I am laughing…"
Zora Neale Hurston

A.   RELEASE Matters

RELEASE…the word itself makes Us relax a little. RELEASE…a concept that makes Us think of freedom, a concept in itself that has special significance for Us. Despite being free of the bonds of slavery, the *legacy* of slavery subjects us to an unusually high amount of *dis*tress and tension on a daily basis.[26] It then becomes unusually important for Us to RELEASE and free Ourselves as much as possible from these negative effects of stress. Unfortunately, the accumulation of tension in Our bodies over time *with little to no RELEASE* is a key source of the unusually high levels of chronic *dis*ease and *dis*tress in Our community. Practice makes perfect, and, with RELEASING, this is also true. RELEASING regularly, especially at times when We don't "need" it, protects Our bodies and minds from stress buildup and creation of unnecessary stress,[27] real MBB! When We RELEASE, We experience the freedom and recovery specifically critical to Our wellbeing!

---

[26] Smith, Clint. "Racism, Stress and Black Death." The New Yorker (16 Jul 2016). *http://www.newyorker.com/news/news-desk/racism-stress-and-black-death*

[27] "Relaxation, Stress and Sleep," Dartmouth Student Wellness Center, *http://www.dartmouth.edu/~healthed/relax/*

B. On the RELEASE TIP

So how do We **GET A GGRiPP** and RELEASE? Laughter!
Simply put, We need to laugh more, until We "bust a gut" daily!
Laughter, especially gut-busting laughter, is one of the most
effective approaches to RELEASE, relaxation and recovery. It is
well known to be the "best medicine" for physical health, relieving
the stress response, lowering the level of stress hormones and
blood pressure, releasing endorphins and relaxing muscles.[28] And,
laughter has always specifically benefited Our mental health; in
fact, We have a cultural tradition of using humor to RELEASE.
Specifically, Our brand of (Black) humor has been an effective
approach We have used consistently to "keep from crying," as an
emotional healing "balm" for "pent up aggression" and also as a
"rich source of creative energy" and a way of "affirming Our
humanity."[29]

Who doesn't love to laugh? When I bust a gut (and crack up), I
notice that I am more "present," experiencing freedom from all
else *in that moment,* forgetting everything except the source of my
laughter. When We laugh, in that funny moment, We are free from
worry (about the future) and regret (about the past). Our mental
state improves and We are better able to deal with negative
situations (and people). Studies show that We laugh primarily
during social interactions[30] (doubling the common-unity effect). In
addition, Black humor has historically given Us a forum for
"elevating the conversation, messaging inspiration, and increasing
the discussion", as well as the "hope and optimism to cope with

---

[28] "Stress relief from laughter? It's no joke." Mayo Clinic, Healthy Lifestyle, Stress Management. (21 Apr 2016). *http://www.mayoclinic.org/healthy-lifestyle/stress-management/in-depth/stress-relief/art-20044456*

[29] Early, G. Carpio, G. and Sollors, W. "Black Humor: Reflections on and American Tradition." Bulletin of the American Academy of Arts & Sciences, (2010): 33-34. *https://www.amacad.org/publications/bulletin/summer2010/humor.pdf*

[30] Martin, Rod A. "Do Children Laugh Much More Often Than Adults Do?" The Association for Applied and Therapeutic Humor. *http://www.aath.org/do-children-laugh-much-more-often-than-adults-do*

difficult times."[31]   So, **GET A GGRiPP** on your "best medicine" and "bust a gut" right now!

1. (T)ype

Laughter! Actively look for those things that make you laugh and RELEASE every day, multiple times a day! It's that simple!

2. (I)ntensity

(Start) Low:

If you haven't RELEASED through laughter much at all lately, start by simply smiling more. Smiling has similar MBB to laughter so start there.

(Go) High:

Want (or need) to RELEASE even more? Turn that :-) into an LOL! Really laugh out loud...and long...as often as possible ...bust a gut!!!

3. (P)ointers

(1) Do a laughter audit and be aware of how many times a day you have a good old-fashioned "gut-busting" laugh! Once you know your starting place, try to add to that number every day! (One study suggests that adults generally laugh less than 20 times a day.[32] If you are the type that likes a target, set that as your daily goal!)

---

[31] Yerman, Marcia G. "Exploring Why We Laugh: Black Comedians on Black Comedy." Huffingtonpost.com (25 May 2011). *http://www.huffingtonpost.com/marcia-g-yerman/why-we-laugh-black-comedi_b_469815.html*

[32] Martin, Rod & A. Kuiper, Nicholas. (1999). "Daily occurrence of laughter: Relationships with age, gender, and Type A personality." Humor - International Journal of Humor Research. 12: 355-384. *https://www.researchgate.net/publication/269621027_Daily_occurrence_of_laughter_Relationships_with_age_gender_and_Type_A_personality*

(2) Since the chances of laughter increase in social situations, intentionally schedule and spend more time around a laughter buddy (or 2 or 4) that shares your sense of humor!

(3) Did you know that even if We don't feel it and "force" laughter (make Ourselves laugh),[33] We can still reap the MBB? In other words, with or without the feeling, We can use laughter (or even a smile) to make Our brains think We feel better (happier).[34] And, generally, it will help the genuine feeling shortly follow!

(4) Need a quick, gut-busting RELEASE? Check out getaggripp.com/release for a variety of great Black comedy links!

---

[33] Eurich, Tasha. "Laughter: The Surprising Secret to Surviving Tough Times." Huffingtonpost.com (5 Oct 2014). *http://www.huffingtonpost.com/tasha-eurich-phd/laughter-the-surprising-s_b_5651354.html*

[34] Wenner, Melinda. "Smile! It Could Make You Happier." Scientific American Mind (1 Sep 2009). *https://www.scientificamerican.com/article/smile-it-could-make-you-happier/*

IV. POWER: Soul Train

> "With the power of soul, anything is possible."
> Jimi Hendrix

A.   POWER Matters

Anyone familiar with Our history knows that "resistance" has always been a necessary part of Our tradition, and not just physically. As We continue to "push" for progress, it is important for Us to "resistance train." "Resistance training" has always been about training one's self in such a way as to increase POWER. Success in resistance (or strength) training is achieved when POWER – defined as the amount of strength and force one can exert - increases. Strength training is also referred to as "resistance training." Increasing the amount of strength and force one can exert with both mind *and* body is especially necessary for Us as racism and oppression takes its toll mentally and physically.[35] Therefore, resistance training (and increasing both physical and mental POWER) is critical in enabling Us to meet the physical *and* mental challenges We confront every day.

Resistance training simultaneously trains Us physically and mentally. By training, We are ultimately teaching our bodies and minds to become POWERful, increasing confidence in Our ability to meet physical and mental challenges. This decreases Our stress when confronted with *new* challenges. Other health and wellness programs incorporate resistance training because it is vital to the

---

[35] "Discrimination Linked to Increased Stress, Poorer Health, American Psychological Association Survey Finds." American Psychological Association (10 Mar 2016). *http://www.apa.org/news/press/releases/2016/03/impact-of-discrimination.aspx*

body. **GET A GGRiPP**'s POWER element reminds Us that resistance training, plays an important role, not just for its ability to develop strong *bodied* individuals but also for its MBB, inspiring a strong *minded*, strong *hearted* and strong *"soul"ed* community.

B.   On the **POWER TIP**

So how do We **GET A GGRiPP** on POWER? A concept unique to **GET A GGRiPP** - "SOUL TRAINing." In other words, the **GET A GGRiPP** approach to POWER makes "training" work uniquely for Us by combining it with "soul." What is "SOUL TRAINing?" **GET A GGRiPP's** SOUL TRAINing combines classic POWER resistance training with "soul line dancing" to create the kind of dance/"work" We can have fun putting in. Like many uniquely African-American cultural customs, "soul line dancing" is an example of how We have used Our "soul"-full culture to create an innovative variation on traditional line dancing.[36] "Soul," or urban, line dancing" is a Black cultural evolution of line dancing, incorporating Our forms of music (i.e. soul, R&B and hip-hop) and accompanying dance steps. SOUL TRAINing takes soul/urban line dancing to the next level for Our health.

As a dance and dance fitness instructor, I have always known and taught exercise "in disguise." SOUL TRAINing does just that, combining dance movements that train the same muscles as traditional fitness exercises in the style of soul line dancing! And, just like with soul line dancing, individual style can be added based on fitness level; you can create or pick low, medium or high intensity variations. At the highest SOUL TRAINing levels, even the most fit folks can "feel the burn." With POWER soul line dancing, We can resistance train and build our POWER using Our soul at a level *We choose*! When We say **"GET A GGRiPP** on POWER," We mean "SOUL TRAINing!"

---

[36] The New Encyclopedia of Southern Culture: Volume 16: Sports and Recreation, p. 141

1. (T)ype

SOUL TRAINing, aka POWER Soul Line Dancing, a POWERful integration of classic strength/resistance training moves with soul/urban line dancing.

2. (I)ntensity

(Start) Low:
Start sLOW, adding one POWER (resistance) move to your soul line dance, using bodyweight only. sLOW moves ensure using muscles (NOT momentum) to build POWER. sLOW moves also allow you to focus on form and correct execution.

(Go) High:
If you want to POWER up, add more strength moves, get up higher, get down lower, add weights or speed it up. Going at a higher Intensity (or intervals, i.e. alternating high and low intensities) requires much more control as you are moving at a faster pace and/or incorporating additional resistance for increased benefit.

3. (P)ointers

(1) Easy POWER (resistance) moves to incorporate for SOUL TRAINing: squats/lunges, pushups/planks, presses, curls.

(2) Before SOUL TRAINing, do at least 3-5 minutes of warmup (dynamic movements) before and at least 3-5 minutes of (static) stretching after.

(3) SOUL TRAINing requires rest for muscles to recover, repair and rebuild. Especially if you use more than your own bodyweight, do your SOUL TRAINing on alternate days with at least 48 hours between SOUL TRAINing sessions.

(4) Remember, the goal is to increase POWER; don't be shy about challenging yourself!

(5) Keep in mind, it's still a dance so add your own unique style and use music that inspires YOU!

(6) Experience SOUL TRAINing POWER Soul Line Dances at getaggripp.com/power!

V. PEACE: Breathe Inside Out

> "If you cannot find peace within yourself, you will
> never find it anywhere else."
> Marvin Gaye

A. PEACE Matters

PEACE is freedom from conflict, pain or anxiety, it is the absence of worry, it is feeling safe and protected. Unfortunately, Our communities are (still) uniquely subject to conflict-ridden, painful, anxiety-inducing, worrisome, "security-threatening" situations (police brutality, white supremacist/KKK/Neo-Nazi, mass incarceration, discrimination, etc.). When We feel conflict, pain, anxiety, worry, insecurity or distress, Our bodies reflect that. We may feel shallow breathing or muscle tension. Unfortunately, shallow breathing leads to lack of oxygen to muscles and other tissue, including Our brains. We are then unable to think clearly or focus. And a vicious cycle begins. To break the cycle, We must learn to trigger what is called "the relaxation response."[37] Long term, triggering this consistently can help Us experience not only better health but also an improved ability to think through and solve problems. While We can't avoid them, We can transform these situations and reduce the effect of distressing situations on Our individual health and the health of Our communities. "Relaxation training" is the practice of "relaxation techniques" to trigger the relaxation response." Just as We **GET A GGRiPP** on POWER through SOUL TRAINing; We **GET A GGRiPP** on PEACE through relaxation training. Relaxation training will

---

[37] Marksberry, Kellie. "Take A Deep Breath." The American Institute of Stress. *https://www.stress.org/take-a-deep-breath/*

enable Us to reap relaxation response MBB, both short term (e.g. relaxed muscles, better mood, clearer thinking) and long term (i.e. improved community health and more effective community solutions).

B.   On the **PEACE TIP**

So how do We **GET A GGRiPP** on PEACE? It starts from within…with a breath. To find PEACE in Our outer environments, We must first find Our inner PEACE.[38]

After dedicating myself consistently to quiet, PEACEful time every day for the last year, I have noticed a significant increase in my feelings of PEACE, calm and overall wellbeing. In fact, I can say with certainty that it has helped me view things more positively ("glass half full") and successfully attract more positive opportunities in my life ("the secret"). There is a saying that "You can't change what's going on around you until you start changing what's going on within you." Only when We find PEACE inside can We bring PEACE to Our outside experiences, effectively moving peace "inside out." We must find more opportunities to **GET A GGRiPP** on PEACE and breathe…deeply. In this way, We can breathe PEACE inside out.

GET A GGRiPP focuses on the breath because deep breathing is the simplest way to trigger the relaxation response but this same result can also come with other approaches or techniques. Acknowledging that Our faith plays such an important role for many in Our community, prayer is another way to reap the same MBB. There are also formal meditation practices such as repeated mantras or affirmations. Whether prayer, mantra, affirmation, or simple deep breathing, work whatever works for you to achieve inner PEACE, breathing what is inside, out!

---

[38] Formica, Michael J. "Change Happens from the Inside." Psychology Today (8 Jan 2010). *https://www.psychologytoday.com/blog/enlightened-living/201001/change-happens-the-inside-out*

1.   (T)ype

BREATHE. DEEP. Inhale slowly. Exhale even more slowly.

2.   (I)ntensity

(Start) Low:

For beginners, start small, 1-2 minutes (or 10-20 breaths) of deep breathing.

(Go) High:

Continue to increase the time you spend deep breathing. Figure out what works best for you. Find two or more times in your day to stop, turn inward, listen to and slow down your breath. If you are the type that likes a target, studies have shown that between 20 and 45 minutes per day can be extremely beneficial. Like your GROOVING, You can also break that time up into morning and evening or more times throughout the day.

3.   (P)ointers

(1) Your mind *will* wander and you may feel restless. This is completely normal; allow thoughts and feelings of restlessness to come and go. Remember, your goal is PEACE, *the absence* of conflict, so don't fight yourself!

(2) Repetition of a word or phrase (mantra, affirmation or prayer) is helpful for triggering the relaxation response. You can use also repeat it to refocus yourself and return your focus to your breath

(3) Identify a space with minimum (little to no) distractions first, where you can practice deep breathing and focusing within. Over time, it will become easier to achieve (inner) PEACE, even with distractions.

(4) Find a comfortable, relaxed position. For some, it is lying down (palms up in receptive mode); others prefer sitting

comfortable cross-legged or with legs out. Sitting positions for meditation and prayer evolved because deep breathing and relaxation may cause you to fall asleep when lying down. If you fall asleep, you probably needed it; remember, this is about PEACE, so don't fight it!!! (also, see Note about SLEEP below)

(5) Adults generally breathe every 3-5 seconds (12-20 breaths per minute). For deep breathing, aim for longer breaths (or fewer breaths per minute). A great target is at least 6 seconds per breath (or less than 10 breaths per minute).

(6) Research shows that triggering the relaxation response is not as effective within 2 hours after a meal.[39] So, do it first thing in the morning, before you eat or wait 2 hours or so after you eat.

(7) To remind yourself to breathe throughout the day, set reminders on your phone, use sticky notes or make it a habit by attaching PEACE and your relaxation training to something you already do (look in the mirror, sit down at your desk) or a place you already go (bathroom, car) regularly.

(8) Guided meditations are helpful to those of Us with very (hyper) active brains. They can support you in your relaxation training using visualization or other techniques. Find suggestions for guided meditations at getaggripp.com/peace!

---

[39] Benson, Herbert M.D., The Relaxation Response, (HarperTorch: 1976): 162-163, http://www.relaxationresponse.org/steps/

ONE MORE THING!

A NOTE ABOUT SLEEP AND *US:* If you were wondering where sleep fits into **GET A GGRiPP**, here it is! Sleep is of course a critical part of overall wellness. Deep breathing, relaxation and stress recovery are automatic benefits of restful sleep. However, many of Us are sleep-deprived. In fact, numerous studies have proven that Black Americans get less sleep on average than other Americans <u>and</u> less of the most effective *recovery phase* of sleep (slow-wave sleep).[40] Knowing that this is not unusual for Us, rather than fight it or beat yourself up (adding to your stress), if increasing sleep time is a challenge for you, perform your deep breathing/PEACE technique at bedtime. Because **GET A GGRiPP** is a "start small, build slowly" solution and PEACE starts within, this will be an easy way to start small *and* it will give you a higher quality sleep for whatever quantity of sleep you *can* get!!

---

[40] "The Racial Inequality of Sleep:" TheAtlantic.com (27 Oct 2015) https://www.theatlantic.com/health/archive/2015/10/the-sleep-gap-and-racial-inequality/412405/

VI. Getting Started

> "Start from where you are.
> Use what you have.
> Do what you can."
> Arthur Ashe

A.   "Start from where you are…"

Remember, making it easy is one of the key factors for success in making healthy lifestyle changes. How you get started is dependent on what will be easiest for you as you "start from where you are." You can…

…keep it simple and begin incorporating whichever **GET A GGRiPP** healthy lifestyle element(s) (GRUB, GROOVE, RELEASE, POWER, PEACE) sounds most enjoyable, easy or interesting to you. Start small, build slow. If an element is new to you, start small by incorporating it once a week for a short period. Or, for variety, start small with a different element every day. Build slowly by gradually doing that element more often or adding new elements, either more times of the day or more days of the week (or both!). Remember, your target is to eventually make habits of all of the GET A GGRiPP elements, incorporating them all every day in a way that is fun and easy for you!

OR

…use the **GET A GGRiPP** Getting Started Questionnaire and Worksheets in the Appendix to identify specific **GET A GGRiPP** element(s) that are easy for you to start on based on where you are currently. Once you have identified the element(s) you want to start with, **GET A GGRiPP** has two methods to support you in incorporating them into your lifestyle: Ease IN and All IN. Although both use the "start small, build slow" approach, The Ease In Method focuses on one **GET A GGRiPP** element at a time and The All-In method encourages you to **GET A GGRiPP** on more than one element at a time. The right method for you depends on your current lifestyle (where you are), your style of learning and what feels manageable, comfortable, accessible and easy for you.

B.   "Use what you have…"

As We have discussed, **GET A GGRiPP** elements are easy and accessible to Us because they "use what We have" and do not require special equipment or memberships. In addition, there is *no more powerful support* in making healthy lifestyle changes *than the social support of Our community*. Research shows "a positive relationship between social support and mental and physical health outcomes"[41] for Us specifically. Research also shows that We "use [Our] informal networks to a greater degree than whites."

All of this points to the *extra*-importance of Our "village!" Find a partner, form a group, share goals and plans, hold each other accountable, support each other in each of the elements, and **GET A GGRiPP** in "Common-unity!" Or join the larger **GET A GGRiPP** Common-Unity online (getaggripp.com, facebook.com/getagripp, #getaggripp on Instagram, Twitter and YouTube)! There, you can find online partners, share your journey and get ongoing information about **GET A GGRiPP** and its healthy lifestyle elements, including resources, tips, info links, quotes, videos, affirminders™, special events and more!

---

[41] Ford, Marvella E., Tilley, Barbara C., and McDonald, Patricia E. "Social Support Among African-American Adults with Diabetes, Part 1: Theoretical Framework." Journal of the National Medical Association, Vol 90, No 6: 363. *https://www.ncbi.nlm.nih.gov/pmc/articles/PMC2568240/pdf/jnma00165-0047.pdf*

C. "Do what you can…"

Although **GET A GGRiPP** encourages Us to **GET A GGRiPP** together in "common-unity," it is also rooted in a culture that thrives on uniqueness, creativity and innovation. So, make it yours! That means…

"Perfectly imperfect"

There is no perfect or right way to **GET A GGRiPP**! Your GGRiPP may need to look slightly different from someone else's in order to make it work for you. **GET A GGRiPP** is all about sharing common cultural aspects while embracing the uniqueness that makes each one of Us special!

"Your pace is the right pace"

You don't have to go in any order. Start with the **GET A GGRiPP** healthy lifestyle element(s) that are easy for you to add, you are most comfortable with or feel you most need or are motivated to do. Do what makes sense for or feels best to you.

"Make small changes now to see big changes later"

Any change is stressful. Don't bite off too much at any one time. Make small changes and allow them to become habits before you make more. Build on small successes to create larger impact.

"Fill the glass half full"

Focusing on positive rather than negative changes enables greater success with lifestyle changes. By focusing changes primarily on adding, - i.e. more grooving, better grub, greater release, increased peace, more power - We increase Our likelihood of successfully changing habits long-term.

"The link is what you think"

Your thoughts and beliefs can create your reality. Believe in yourself, the power of Our roots and the strength of Our cultural legacy! **GET A GGRiPP** on any negative self-talk. If you believe it, you can achieve it!

D.   "Track your progress..."

"If you can't fly, then run.
If you can't run, then walk.
If you can't walk, then crawl.
But whatever you do, you have to keep moving
forward."
Martin Luther King Jr.

Along with Our targeted health and wellness plan, We need methods of tracking Our progress that are supportive of Us, providing a sense of progress and success without creating unnecessary stress. A common method of measuring health status, scales and BMI charts can be misleading, specifically for Us.[42] And, of course, We should keep it simple to prevent unnecessary stress (don't stress or obsess!). **GET A GGRiPP** suggests:

> If overall health improvement is your goal, know your numbers. That is, check the following 3 items regularly (see below for an example of a quarterly tracker of these three numbers) and track your progress.
> 1. blood pressure (ideally <=120/80)
> 2. blood glucose (sugar) (ideally <100mg/dL fasting or <6% A1C)
> 3. and cholesterol (ideally < 200mg/dL total; with HDL> 40 and LDL<130)
>
> These tests are simple and can be done at local drugstores, health clinics and other facilities as well as community health fairs. The key, however, is in getting treated if it is below the ideal targets (or above for

---

[42] "Ethnic Differences in BMI and Disease Risk." Harvard University, TH Chan School of Public Health. *https://www.hsph.harvard.edu/obesity-prevention-source/ethnic-differences-in-bmi-and-disease-risk/*

LDL) mentioned above. Regular and consistent tracking is important and treatment is critical; especially in the case of blood pressure, a "silent killer" in Our community.

Overall Health Measures	Q1	Q2	Q3	Q4
Blood Pressure				
Blood Glucose				
Cholesterol				

If weight loss and/or fat loss and muscle gain are your goal, keep it simple. Check the following item (see below for an example of a quarterly tracker) and track your progress.

1. waist measurement

Your waist measurement can give you a good sense of your weight progress and health risk and can be "more accurate compared to BMI" for health risk predictions.[43] Get a tape measure and measure around your waist midway between the top of your hip bone and the bottom of your ribs. Check it 2 or 3 times for accuracy. … Generally, if you want to "whittle your waist" *and* lower your health risk, work towards a

---

[43] Kekatos, Mary. "Hip-to-waist ratio is far better than BMI at measuring your health: Study says people carrying an 'extra tire' have far more problems - whether they're skinny or fat." DailyMail.com (26 Apr 2017). *http://www.dailymail.co.uk/health/article-4448060/Hip-waist-ratio-important-BMI-study-says.html*

number of less than 35 in (88 cm) for women and less than 40 in (102 cm) for men.[44]

Weight Loss/Fat Loss and Muscle Gain Measures	Q1	Q2	Q3	Q4
Waist size				

The easiest option to track weight loss and/or fat loss and muscle gain? Find a piece of clothing that can be your personal measure of progress. Clothes don't lie!!!

---

[44] "Waist size matters in diagnosing obesity among minorities." American Heart Association (9 Jul 2015). *http://news.heart.org/waist-size-matters-in-diagnosing-obesity-among-minorities/*

ONE MORE THING!

A NOTE ABOUT HEALTHCARE AND <u>US</u>: **GET A GGRiPP** is based on the premise that Our outcomes, health (and other-wise) are stronger when We work together *in community*. When it comes to the (US) healthcare system, We can and *should* use a similar approach. Given the prevalence of discrimination, bias against and, in certain cases, outright abuse of Black patients, We are often (justifiably) distrustful of doctors and hospitals. Institutional racism in the US healthcare system is real[45]; however, We *have* to know Our health status in order to know what we need to do to improve it and **GET A GGRiPP**. We *must* meet our immediate needs (i.e. diagnosis and, as necessary, treatment) using the existing system, even as We work to improve the system. How? First, in community, we should share with each other (choose) and support doctors, hospitals and facilities that have positive outcomes with Black patients. Second, We can educate Ourselves, support each other *and* focus on facts and numbers. Unlike discrimination, facts (e.g. symptoms of

---

[45] Schroeder, Michael O. " Racial Bias in Medicine Leads to Worse Care for Minorities." US News & World Report, usnews.com (11 Feb 2016). *http://health.usnews.com/health-news/patient-advice/articles/2016-02-11/racial-bias-in-medicine-leads-to-worse-care-for-minorities*

heart attack, stroke, diabetes) and numbers (e.g. blood pressure, blood glucose) are unbiased and will support us in doing what We need to do to reach Our goals.

OUTRO

Wellness MATTERS.

In order for Us to finally achieve Our goals for both health and wellness *and* social and racial progress, We need a *culturally-rooted*, *culturally-targeted*, mind *and* body WELLNESS solution that represents *Us*. **We need GET A GGRIPP** (2G's, 1R, 2P's). **GET A GGRiPP** represents a new approach to wellness specifically for peoples of African descent. Targeting Our unique needs for both mind and body, **GET A GGRiPP** is the "for Us, by Us" health and wellness solution that helps Us succeed by focusing on activities that are easy, accessible and fun "for Us" and rooted in traditions "by Us." More than a plan, **GET A GGRiPP** is a health and wellness movement that will help Us 1) improve Our health outcomes **and** 2) create a HEALTHIER, STRONGER Common-Unity foundation for continued social and racial progress!

To borrow a phrase from John and Russell Rickford, authors of Spoken Soul, "we must begin to do for [health] what we have done historically... for our hair, our clothes, our art, our education, and our religion…"[46] That is, We must bring the same cultural roots, determination, style, soul and imperative to Our health that We bring to everything else! How? By bringing cultural determination to each bite (gettin' that green in Our GRUB), bringing cultural roots to each step (showin' Our roots with Our GROOVE), bringing cultural style to each laugh (bustin' a gut in Our RELEASE), bringing cultural soul to each lift (soul trainin' for Our POWER) and bringing a cultural imperative to each breath (breathin' inside out to Our PEACE).

---

[46] Rickford, John Russell and Rickford, Russell John. "In Praise of Spoken Soul." Stanford Magazine (Sept/Oct 2000): 75. *https://alumni-gsb.stanford.edu/get/page/magazine/article/?article_id=40040*

So... what will you do differently starting today...?

You can...

>...eat more green and grub better!
>...dance harder and groove more!
>...laugh louder and release more!
>...resistance train with soul and power up!
>...breathe deeper and peace out!

Remember, the principle is that it will be *easier* for you to form *these* healthy lifestyle habits...because they are rooted in what you already know.

With each bite, step, laugh, lift and breath, We *will* finally **GET A GGRiPP** on what has had a grip on Us for far too long...

GET A...

GRUB: Get That Green

GROOVE: Show Your Roots

RELEASE: Bust a Gut

i

POWER: Soul Train

PEACE: Breathe Inside Out

Postface

Me: Are you experiencing any of these symptoms, Magnus?"

Magnus: "Yes, I am. What does it mean?"

Me: "It means we need to get you to a doctor…*now.*"

Unfortunately, that's not how my conversation with Magnus went - for any number of reasons: because I didn't want to pry, because I didn't want to be pushy, because he was a grown ass man. Whatever the reason, none was a good one for *not having the conversation,* especially when compared to the possible outcome from *having it:* he would still be with us today. As GET A GGRiPP helps Us all take a step toward improved community health awareness, support and prevention, here's "one more thing" to support Us in *having the conversation* I wish I had had with Magnus.

ONE MORE THING!

A NOTE ABOUT HEART DISEASE AND <u>US</u>: According to the American Heart Association, Black Americans are disproportionately affected by **obesity** and **diabetes** *and* have the highest prevalence of **high blood pressure** *in the world.*[47] This means that We suffer uniquely from **the three most**

---

[47] "African Americans and Heart Disease, Stroke." American Heart Association (Jul 2015). http://www.heart.org/HEARTORG/Conditions/More/MyHeartandStrokeNews/African-Americans-and-Heart-Disease_UCM_444863_Article.jsp

common conditions that increase the risk of heart disease. In order for Us to GET A GGRiPP on heart disease (and preventable deaths like Magnus'), as We implement the healthy lifestyle elements of GET A GGRiPP, We can become educated and aware of the signs and symptoms of potentially fatal heart disease conditions. Remember these symptoms…

PAIN: Where? Although chest pain is the most common symptom, you may not experience it or experience it mildly, especially women, **who experience symptoms differently than men**. Pain can also occur in the arm, shoulder, neck and jaw.

INDIGESTION-LIKE SYMPTOMS: Less common symptoms include indigestion, lack of appetite and nausea/vomiting. In fact, these symptoms are often mistaken for indigestion/acid reflux.

FLU-LIKE SYMPTOMS: Often mistaken for the flu, other less common symptoms include wheezing or coughing (especially with white or pink mucus), cold sweats, lightheadedness or fainting and shortness of breath.

SWELLING: Fluid retention is common, especially in the lower extremities, i.e. feet, ankles, legs, abdomen.

PREMONITION: Your heart may race and you may feel severe anxiety, confusion or even a sense of "doom."

YOU ARE NOT JUST TIRED; DON'T GO TO SLEEP! Fatigue and tiredness are also common. If you experience more than one of these symptoms, see a medical professional *immediately*, *especially* if you have high blood pressure.

Appendix 1. GET A GGRiPP Getting Started Questionnaire

The **GET A GGRiPP** Getting Started Questionnaire is designed to help you figure out which **GET A GGRiPP** element(s) (GRUB, GROOVE, RELEASE, POWER, PEACE) you should start with. Remember, We want to make things easy and accessible, starting small and building slowly to successfully make healthy, lasting lifestyle changes. In order to succeed, it is important that We "start from where We are." The **GET A GGRiPP** Getting Started questionnaire will help you figure out which elements might be "quick wins" for you based on two key factors for success. The two key factors are

1) EASE (how easy it will be to make that element a part of your lifestyle)

and

2) HEALTH BENEFIT (how much added benefit that element can provide to your health).

The **GET A GGRiPP** Getting Started questionnaire is intended to help you define these two key factors for your, current unique situation and lifestyle, i.e. based on "where you are." An element's EASE score on the questionnaire reflects how easy that element might be for you based on your current level of enjoyment, ability and interest. An element's HEALTH BENEFIT score reflects the potential additional health benefit for you given what you already do around that element.

Questionnaire Instructions

Calculate an EASE and HEALTH BENEFIT score <u>for each element</u> (GRUB, GROOVE, RELEASE, POWER, PEACE) following the instructions below.

STEP 1:

    Score your answer to the HEALTH BENEFIT question:

      a) If your answer is Yes, give yourself a score of 0 points. (There will be less additional benefit because you already do a lot in this area!)

      b) If you are "almost" a Yes, give yourself a score of 1 point.

      c) If you "do a 'lil something'," give yourself a score of 2 points.

      d) If your answer is No, give yourself a score of 3 points.

STEP 2:

    Score your answer to the EASE questions (Enjoyment, Ability and Interest) questions:

      a) For each Yes answer, give yourself 3 points.

      b) For each No answer, give yourself 0 points.

STEP 3:

    Calculate your total HEALTH BENEFIT score and your total EASE score <u>for that element only</u>.

STEP 4:

    Go to the next element and repeat Steps 1-3.

Remember, when complete, you should have 5 different HEALTH BENEFIT and EASE scores, one for each **GET A GGRiPP** healthy lifestyle element.

GET A GGRiPP
GETTING STARTED QUESTIONNAIRE:

GRUB – Get That Green

Health Benefit	Do you currently eat at least 3 servings/day or 20 servings/week of green leafy vegetables?	
GRUB Score - HEALTH BENEFIT:		
Enjoyment	1) Do you like green leafy vegetables?	
Ability	2) Is it easy for you to make recipes with or get access to green leafy vegetables?	
Interest	3) Do you want to eat more green leafy vegetables?	
GRUB Score - EASE:		

GROOVE – Show Your Roots

Health Benefit	Do you currently dance at least 30 minutes/day or 150 minutes/week at a moderate or vigorous intensity?	
GROOVE Score – HEALTH BENEFIT:		
Enjoyment	1) Do you like to dance?	
Ability	2) Is it easy to convince you to dance?	
Interest	3) Do you want to dance more?	
GROOVE Score - EASE:		

RELEASE – Bust… a Gut

Health Benefit	Do you currently laugh at least 15 times/day?	
RELEASE Score – HEALTH BENEFIT:		
Enjoyment	1) Do you like to laugh?	
Ability	2) Is it easy for you to laugh?	
Interest	3) Do you want to laugh more?	
RELEASE Score - EASE:		

(Getting Started Questionnaire cont'd)

POWER – Soul Train

Health Benefit	Do you currently strength or resistance train for at least 15 minutes/day 2 times/week?	
POWER Score – HEALTH BENEFIT:		
Enjoyment	1) Do you like to strength train?	
Ability	2) Is it easy for you to strength train?	
Interest	3) Do you want to strength train (more)?	
POWER Score - EASE:		

PEACE – Breathe Inside Out

Health Benefit	Do you currently practice a relaxation technique (breathing, mantra, affirmation, and/or prayer) at least 20 minutes/day?	
PEACE Score – HEALTH BENEFIT:		
Enjoyment	1) Do you like quiet and stillness?	
Ability	2) Is it easy for you to be quiet and still?	
Interest	3) Do you want to start/increase a relaxation practice (breathing, mantra, affirmation, and/or prayer)?	
PEACE Score - EASE:		

Evaluating your Scores

STEP 1:

Make a list the element(s) where your HEALTH BENEFIT Score is 2 or 3. These are the element(s) you should focus on to start (because they can benefit you most).

a) If there is only one element, that is your element to focus on. Go straight to STEP 3.

b) If there are <u>no</u> elements with a HEALTH BENEFIT Score of 2 or 3, make your list instead using elements with a HEALTH BENEFIT Score of 1.

STEP 2:

Sort your list of elements from STEP 1 based on EASE score from highest to lowest (highest score first). You should start working on the element(s) with the highest EASE score(s) (especially with scores of 6 or higher) because they will most likely be the easiest to incorporate in your current lifestyle.

STEP 3:

Choose a method: Ease IN or All IN. (see Appendix 2) Depending on the number of elements you plan to focus on (1-5), either method will work. The following are suggestions for which method to choose depending on how many elements in your list from Step 1.

a) If you plan to focus on 1 element (for example, GRUB only), use the Ease IN method and focus on that element for at least a month.

b) If you plan to focus on 2-3 elements, use the Ease IN method and use a weekly period OR use a modified All IN method with only those 2 or 3 elements.

c) if you plan to focus on 4-5 elements, use the Ease IN method and use a daily period OR use the All IN method with your elements of focus.

Take the **GET A GGRiPP** Getting Started Questionnaire periodically and post your results somewhere you can see them. Even better, share your scores and plan (see below) with a partner or health buddy. Your target is a HEALTH BENEFIT score of 0 and an EASE score of 9 for *every* **GET A GGRiPP** healthy lifestyle element. Getting there means that you are getting all the health benefit you can and you have a great GGRiPP on the keys to wellness. Keep doing what you are doing, ideally while supporting others in getting there too!

Appendix 2. GET A GGRiPP Planning: Ease IN and All IN

Now that you have decided on your element(s) of focus, you are ready to start incorporating the **GET A GGRiPP** healthy lifestyle elements into your daily life: As listed below, there are two methods to support planning **GET A GGRiPP** lifestyle changes: Ease IN and All IN. Although both use the "start small, build slow" approach, The Ease In Method focuses on one **GET A GGRiPP** element at a time and The All-In method encourages you to **GET A GGRiPP** on more than one element at a time. The right method for you depends on your current lifestyle (where you are), your style of learning and what feels best for you. Here are a few things to keep in mind as you get started with the planning methods:

- Although the instructions and samples provided are for daily or weekly periods, **you should choose whatever period you believe will work best for you** – literally, "it's all good" when it comes to **GET A GGRiPP**! You are building habits so take your time to build them right! Also, whichever period you choose, start on a day (like Sunday) when you will most likely have the free time to allocate to creating your first small success!

- Remember, "start from where you are." Use the TIPs to find your level and determine your target intensity and approach for the day (or week depending on your focus): low, high, or anywhere in between. Adjust your target intensity up or down. Here are sample daily and weekly targets for each healthy lifestyle element:

GET A GGRiPP Healthy Lifestyle Element	Beginner Target (Low)	Advanced Target (High)
GRUB: Get that Green	1 serving (cup) leafy greens/day	5-10 servings (cups) leafy greens/day
GROOVE: Show Your Roots	10 dancing* minutes/day	60 minutes/day (6 units) or 300 minutes/week dancing*
RELEASE: Bust a Gut	1 (Kool-Aid) smile or gut-busting laugh/day	20 gut-busting laughs/day
POWER: Soul Train	10 minutes/week	30 minutes/3 times/week**
PEACE: Breathe Inside Out	5 minutes deep breathing/day	20-45 minutes deep breathing/day

*moderate intensity (can talk, can't sing)
**over 2 or 3 days

GET A GGRiPP
Ease IN Planning Method:

The "Ease IN" method helps you plan to improve your intensity on one **GET A GGRiPP** element at a time. Once you have chosen the element(s) you want to focus on to start (by choosing elements that sound easy and accessible to you or using the Getting Started questionnaire above), pick your "Ease In" period. For example, "Easing in" daily means you will assign a focus element to each day of the week. Easing in weekly means you will focus on one element for an entire week before moving on to another element.

Ease IN Daily instructions: Assign an element of focus to a day of the week. Set a starting target intensity for that element. Set your target intensity based on what will make you successful, something easy and accessible for you. Each day, focus on the assigned element and meeting the target intensity level. Adjust your target intensity up or down as needed.

Ease IN Weekly instructions: Assign an element of focus to a week. Set a starting target intensity for that element. Set your target intensity based on what will make you successful, something easy and accessible for you. Every day of that week, focus on the assigned element and meeting the target intensity level. Adjust your target intensity up or down as needed.

SAMPLE "Ease IN" Plan (Daily):

Day of the Week	Element of Focus	Approach (How much and when)
Sunday	PEACE	"Breathe inside out" for 5 minutes this morning
Monday	GRUB	"Get that green", at least one serving at one meal
Tuesday	PEACE	"Breathe inside out" for 5 minutes this evening
Wednesday	GRUB	"Get that green", at least one serving at one meal
Thursday	POWER	"Soul train" for 5 minutes this morning or evening
Friday	RELEASE	"Bust a gut" at least 5 times during the day
Saturday	GROOVE	"Show your roots" for 5 minutes this evening

SAMPLE "Ease IN" Plan (Weekly):

Week (Dates)	Element of Focus	Approach (How much and when)
Week 1 (Jul 1-7)	PEACE	"Breathe inside out" for 5 minutes this evening
Week 2 (Jul 8-14)	GRUB	"Get that green", at least one serving at one meal
Week 3 (Jul 15-21)	POWER	"Soul train" for 5 minutes this morning or evening
Week 4 (Jul 22-28)	RELEASE	"Bust a gut" at least 5 times during the day
Week 5 (Jul 29-Aug 4)	GROOVE	"Show your roots" for 5 minutes this evening

"Ease IN" Planning Worksheet

Day of the Week or Week (with Dates)	Healthy Lifestyle Element of Focus	Approach (Target intensity: Low or High, How much? How many times? How many minutes?)	Notes (How did I do? What was easiest? What was hardest? How can I adjust for greater success?)

GET A GGRiPP
All IN Planning Method:

The "All IN" method helps you plan to improve your intensity on many (or all) elements simultaneously; since you are incorporating many elements at one time, it is more complex than Ease IN. See the sample "All IN" scorecard below. You can set and track your target intensities for your focus elements (see sample targets above). For each element, pick a daily or weekly target intensity and use the checkboxes to track your progress. For example, the sample scorecard has a 30-minute daily intensity target for Groove. Because the checkbox unit is 10 minutes; when 30 minutes is completed, 3 checkboxes would be checked. You can choose the unit for each checkbox (see the sample scorecard for suggestions).

SAMPLE "All IN" Plan and Scorecard (Weekly):

GET A GGRiPP healthy lifestyle element	Target Intensity					
GRUB (unit: 1 serving)	5 servings	☐	☐	☐	☐	☐
GROOVE (unit: 10 minutes)	30 minutes	☐	☐	☐		
RELEASE (unit: 1 gut-busting laugh)	5 laughs	☐	☐	☐	☐	☐
POWER (unit: 10 minutes)	10 minutes	☐				
PEACE (unit: 5 minutes breathing)	5 minutes	☐	☐	☐	☐	☐

"All IN" Planning Worksheet and Scorecard:

GET A GGRiPP healthy lifestyle element _Target Intensity_	GRUB (checkbox unit: ___ serving greens) ___ servings	GROOVE (checkbox unit: ___ minutes) ___ minutes	RELEASE (checkbox unit: ___ gut-busting laugh) ___ laughs	POWER (checkbox unit: ___ minutes) ___ minutes	PEACE (checkbox unit: ___ minutes of breathing) ___ minutes
☐	☐	☐	☐	☐	☐
☐	☐	☐	☐	☐	☐
☐	☐	☐	☐	☐	☐
☐	☐	☐	☐	☐	☐
☐	☐	☐	☐	☐	☐
☐	☐	☐	☐	☐	☐
☐	☐	☐	☐	☐	☐
☐	☐	☐	☐	☐	☐
☐	☐	☐	☐	☐	☐
☐	☐	☐	☐	☐	☐

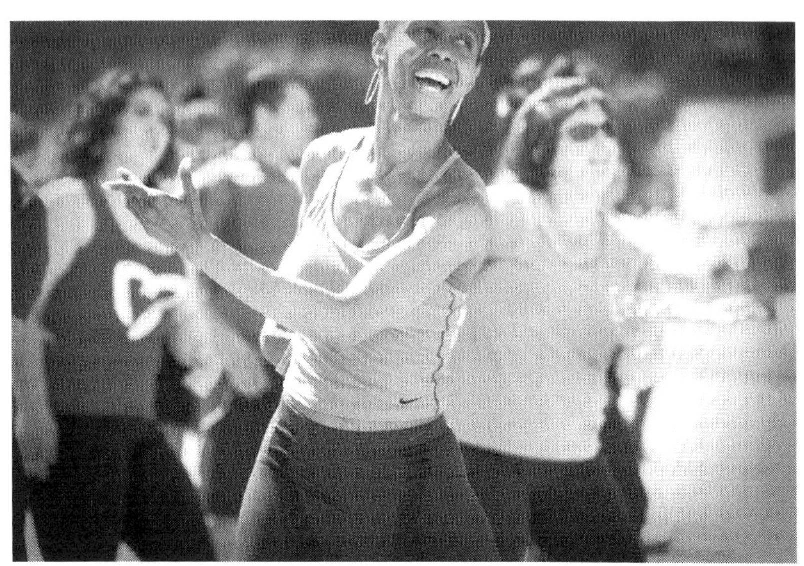

About Tanya

Tanya Leake is a passionate student and teacher of wellness principles, committed to supporting others in re/discovering *their* best, healthiest selves and practicing what she preaches. After 18 years as a senior business strategy and technology consultant, she left corporate America, dedicating herself full-time to supporting others attain lifestyles that "EmBODY WELL."

Using her engineering skills (she earned her Bachelor of Science in Industrial Engineering from Stanford University) and her consulting experience, she developed the precursor to GET A GGRiPP, the "EmBODY WELL" framework, designed to support individuals in embodying their personal well/being. A holistic approach guides her framework's total mind-body focus on physical, mental *and* emotional balance, re/discovery and awareness. Tanya also blogs and speaks about her trademarked vegetablarian™ approach, providing a simpler back-to-basics approach to eating for your health. With an emphasis on practical tools, follow her EmBODY WELL YouTube channel and cook along with Grub and Groove, her vegetablarian cooking show, or dance along with her original dance fitness videos. From her customer-acclaimed WELLshops™ and group dance and fitness classes to her private sessions, she supports groups big and small, private, public and corporate, as well as individuals about the why, what and how to eat, do and embody WELL.

Tanya is a certified ACE (American Council on Exercise) health coach and group fitness instructor, a holistic wellness consultant, trainer and facilitator who specializes in holistic nutrition, self-care, and dance fitness. She holds specialty certificates in women's health, natural health, sports and exercise nutrition and nutrition therapy and is currently pursuing her Master's Degree in Clinical Nutrition. She still performs, dances and teaches regularly in ATL, NY, and the SF Bay Area. For more information or to book Tanya, visit embodywell.com.